INTRODUCTION

Saxenda (liraglutide) is used for weight loss and to help keep weight off once weight has been lost, it's miles used for overweight adults or overweight adults who additionally have weight-associated scientific issues. Saxenda can be used in kids aged 12 to 17 years who with weight problems and who have a bodyweight above 132 pounds (60 kg). Saxenda is used together with a wholesome weight-reduction plan and exercising. Saxenda is an injection given once an afternoon beneath the skin (subcutaneous) from a multi-dose injection pen.

Saxenda contains the identical lively ingredient (liraglutide) as Victoza. The difference among Saxenda and Victoza is they are exceptional strengths and they may be FDA authorised for specific conditions. Saxenda isn't always for treating type 1 or type 2 diabetes. It is not recognised if Saxenda is secure and effective in youngsters below 12 years of age. It is not known if Saxenda is safe and powerful in children elderly 12 to 17 years with kind 2 diabetes.

BEFORE USING SAXENDA

You have to now not use Saxenda in case you are allergic to liraglutide, or if you have:

• A couple of endocrine neoplasia kind 2 (tumors for your glands);

• A personal or family history of medullary thyroid carcinoma (a form of thyroid cancer); or

• Diabetic ketoacidosis (call your doctor for treatment). You ought to no longer use Saxenda if you additionally use insulin or different medicines like liraglutide (albiglutide, dulaglutide, exenatide, Byetta, Bydureon,

Tanzeum, Trulicity). To make sure Saxenda is safe for you, tell your medical doctor when you have:

• belly troubles causing slow digestion;

• Kidney or liver disorder;

• High triglycerides (a form of fats inside the blood);

• Coronary heart problems;

• A records of troubles along with your pancreas or gallbladder; or

• A records of despair or suicidal thoughts.

In animal studies, liraglutide induced thyroid tumors or thyroid cancer. It isn't recognized whether or not these effects would arise in humans the usage of ordinary doses. Ask your medical doctor approximately your danger. It isn't acknowledged whether Saxenda will damage an unborn toddler. Tell your health practitioner in case you are pregnant or plan to grow to be pregnant. It isn't always known whether or not liraglutide passes into breast milk or if it can have an effect on the nursing infant. Tell your physician if you are breast-feeding.

Saxenda isn't FDA-authorised to be used by way of anybody more youthful than 18 years old.

HOW OUGHT TO I USE SAXENDA?

Saxenda is commonly given once in step with day. Follow all guidelines on your prescription label. Your medical doctor may now and again trade your dose. Do now not use this medicine in larger or smaller quantities or for longer than recommended. Do now not use Saxenda and Victoza together. These two brands include the equal energetic aspect but they need to no longer be used together. Read all patient data, remedy guides, and practise sheets provided to you. Ask your doctor or pharmacist when you have any questions. Saxenda is injected beneath the pores and skin at any time of the day, without or with a meal. You will be shown a way to use injections at home. Do no longer self-inject this medicine in case you do not understand the way to deliver the injection and properly cast off used needles and syringes. Saxenda is available in a prefilled injection pen. Ask your pharmacist which kind of needles is exceptional to use along with your pen. Your care provider will display you the best locations in your frame to inject Saxenda. Use distinctive vicinity every time you supply an injection. Do no longer inject into the identical location instances in a row. Do no longer use Saxenda if it has changed colorations or if it has debris in it. Call your pharmacist for brand spanking new medication. Also look ahead to signs and symptoms of high blood sugar (hyperglycemia) including elevated thirst or urination, blurred imaginative and prescient, headache, and tiredness. Blood sugar degrees can be affected by strain, contamination, surgery, exercise, alcohol use, or skipping meals. Ask your medical doctor before changing your dose or remedy time table.

Use a disposable needle simplest once. Follow any state or local laws about throwing away used needles and syringes. Use a puncture-proof "sharps" disposal container (ask your pharmacist in which to get one and the way to throw it away). Keep this field out of the attain of kids and pets. Saxenda is only a part of a whole remedy program that may also consist of diet, exercising, weight manage, regular blood sugar checking out, and special hospital treatment. Follow your health practitioner's commands very intently.

Storing unopened injection pens: Store inside the fridge. Do now not freeze Saxenda, and throw away the medication if it has become frozen. Do no longer use an unopened injection pen if the expiration date on the label has handed. Storing after your first use: You may also maintain "in-use" injection pens in the fridge or at room temperature. Protect the pens from moisture, warmth, and sunlight. Use inside 30 days. Remove the needle earlier than storing an injection pen, and keep the cap at the pen when no longer in use.

Get emergency medical help if you have symptoms of a hypersensitivity to Saxenda: hives; fast heartbeats; dizziness; hassle respiratory or swallowing; swelling of your face, lips, tongue, or throat. Call your medical doctor right away if you have:

• racing or pounding heartbeats;

• Unexpected modifications in temper or behavior, suicidal mind;

• Severe ongoing nausea, vomiting, or diarrhea;

- Signs and symptoms of a thyroid tumor - swelling or a lump on your neck, trouble swallowing, a hoarse voice, feeling quick of breathe;

- Gallbladder problems - fever, top belly pain, clay-colored stools, jaundice (yellowing of your skin or eyes);

- Signs and symptoms of pancreatitis - severe ache in your upper stomach spreading for your back, nausea without or with vomiting, fast heart fee;

- severely low blood sugar - excessive weakness, confusion, tremors, sweating, rapid heart charge, problem speaking, nausea, vomiting, fast respiration, fainting, and seizure (convulsions); or

•	Kidney issues - very little urination; painful or tough urination; swelling on your ft or ankles; feeling worn-out or brief of breath. Common Saxenda facet outcomes may include:

•	Nausea (in particular while you begin using Saxenda), vomiting, stomach ache;

•	Increased heart price;

•	Diarrhea, constipation;

•	Headache, dizziness; or

- Feeling tired.

This isn't always a complete list of facet effects and others might also occur. Call your physician for clinical recommendation about aspect effects. You may also document facet consequences to FDA at 1-800-FDA-1088.

WHAT HAVE TO I TELL MY CARE CREW EARLIER THAN I TAKE THIS MEDICINAL DRUG?

They want to recognise if you have any of these conditions:

- Endocrine tumors (MEN 2) or if someone in your own family had these tumors

- Gallbladder sickness

- High ldl cholesterol

- History of alcohol abuse hassle

- History of pancreatitis

- Kidney ailment or in case you are on dialysis

- Liver ailment

- Previous swelling of the tongue, face, or lips with difficulty breathing, problem swallowing, hoarseness, or tightening of the throat

- Stomach problems

- Suicidal thoughts, plans, or attempt; a previous suicide attempt by you or a member of the family

- Thyroid most cancers or if someone for your circle of relatives had thyroid cancer

- An uncommon or allergic reaction to liraglutide, different medications, meals, dyes, or preservatives

- Pregnant or trying to get pregnant

- Breast-feeding

HOW MUST I USE THIS REMEDY?

This medication is for injection beneath the skin of your higher leg, belly place, or upper arm. You may be taught how to put together and deliver this medicinal drug. Use precisely as directed. Take your medicinal drug at ordinary periods. Do now not take it greater regularly than directed. This remedy comes with INSTRUCTIONS FOR USE. Ask your pharmacist for directions on how to use this medicine. Read the facts carefully. Talk to your pharmacist or care team when you have questions.

It is vital that you positioned your used needles and syringes in a unique sharps field. Do not put them in a trash can. If you do not have a sharps box, name your pharmacist or care team to get one. A unique MedGuide may be given to you by using the pharmacist with every prescription and fill up. Be sure to read this information carefully on every occasion. Talk in your care team approximately the use of this medicine in youngsters. While it can be prescribed for children as young as 12 years of age for decided on situations, precautions do follow.

Overdosage: If you suspect you have taken too much of this remedy contact a poison manipulate middle or emergency room right away. NOTE: This medication is most effective for you. Do no longer percentage this medication with others.

WHAT SHOULD I LOOK AHEAD TO WHILST THE USE OF THIS REMEDY?

Visit your care crew for regular assessments in your progress. Drink plenty of fluids whilst taking this remedy. Check along with your care crew if you get an assault of intense diarrhea, nausea, and vomiting. The loss of too much frame fluid can make it dangerous with a view to take this medicinal drug. This medication may additionally affect blood sugar ranges. Ask your care group if adjustments in food plan or medicines are wished if you have diabetes.

Patients and their households should be careful for worsening depression or thoughts of suicide. Also be careful for sudden adjustments in emotions consisting of feeling traumatic, agitated, panicky, irritable, adversarial, competitive, impulsive, significantly stressed, overly excited and hyperactive, or not being able to sleep. If this happens, especially at the beginning of remedy or after a trade in dose, call your care group. Women have to inform their care crew in the event that they desire to grow to be pregnant or suppose they might be pregnant. Losing weight at the same time as pregnant isn't suggested and can motive harm to the unborn child. Talk in your care group for more information.

WHAT SIDE OUTCOMES CAN ALSO I OBSERVE FROM RECEIVING THIS MEDICINE?

Side consequences that you should record to your care crew as quickly as possible:

• Allergic reactions or angioedema—pores and skin rash, itching, hives, swelling of the face, eyes, lips, tongue, arms, or legs, problem swallowing or respiration

• Fast or abnormal heartbeat

• Gallbladder problems—intense belly pain, nausea, vomiting, and fever

- Kidney harms—decrease in the amount of urine, swelling of the ankles, palms, or feet

- Pancreatitis—severe belly pain that spreads in your again or receives worse after consuming or when touched, fever, nausea, vomiting

- Thoughts of suicide or self-harm, worsening mood, feelings of melancholy

- Thyroid cancer—new mass or lump in the neck, ache or problem swallowing, trouble respiratory, hoarseness

Side results that commonly do no longer require medical attention (file for your care group if they hold or are bothersome):

- Constipation

- Dizziness

- Fatigue

- Headache

- Loss of Appetite

- Nausea

- Upset stomach

This listing might not describe all possible aspect results. Call your medical doctor for medical recommendation about side results. You may also record side results to FDA at 1-800-FDA-1088.

WHAT CAN ALSO INTERACT WITH THIS MEDICINAL DRUG?

• Insulin and different medications for diabetes

This listing might not describe all possible interactions. Give your health care company a list of all the drug treatments, herbs, non-pharmaceuticals, or nutritional supplements you operate. Also inform them in case you smoke, drink alcohol, or use unlawful drugs. Some items may additionally interact together with your medicine.

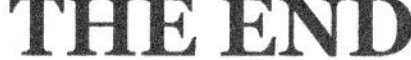

THE END

www.ingramcontent.com/pod-product-compliance
Lightning Source LLC
Chambersburg PA
CBHW071217260726
48653CB00041B/996